THE BEST 10 DAYS OF YOUR LIFE

A Guide to Staying Sane in Trying Times

By Anna Brown

ISBN: 978-0-6489010-1-3

DEDICATION

This book is dedicated to my parents, who gave me all the skills for making a happy life, and to every researcher who has completed the painstaking task of creating a study into the science of happiness.

CONTENTS

CONTENTS

INTRODUCTION

I'm an annoyingly positive person. I sing (badly) in the mornings, and I look forward to getting out of bed every day; I don't have a perfect life – far from it – but I do approach life with the idea that I can enjoy it.

In my early twenties, I spent two years in very poor health, in and out of hospital, and many of the things I enjoyed doing went out the window. I had low energy, couldn't do sport, couldn't stay out late with my friends or generally experience many of the joys of being 20 years old and full of life. I began to empathise with those who struggled with mental health, and to devise ways to experience joy at a slower pace.

Fortunately, my health issues resolved and I'm now able to look back on those darker days with the gift of hindsight – knowing that many of the techniques I naturally used to stay upbeat (with a little loving nagging from my mum perhaps) are scientifically proven ways to get out of a rut.

During my early adulthood, it began to dawn on me that not everybody is an optimist, and that some people experience reality in a very different way from how I perceive those same experiences. This drove me to start a blog named The Happiness Wagon to research the mechanics of happiness. The blog is partly an exploration of why these differences exist, and partly a way to share my own wisdom in cheerfulness, based on lived experience, scientific research and my day job as a health professional.

From there a book was a natural evolution, and I released a short guide on gut health and happiness. Now, with 2020 shaping up to be an interesting year, I figured it's never been a better time to exercise your mental fitness and improve your resilience.

I'll be blunt, ten days isn't enough to magically disappear away your problems, but it is enough to know that you can change your life, or at least your attitude towards it, and ultimately, whether you enjoy the ride. This 10 Day Challenge is a toolbox, not a quick-fix fits-all easy-open solution.

If you've come this far – ordered a book on positivity, cracked it open and actually begun reading – you stand a good chance of having a really good time for the next week and a half, and beyond. If you want a more resilient, fulfilled life, this book is for you.

PREPARATION

Before you start, sit down with a pen and paper, or a blank document on your screen, and think about what exactly you're trying to achieve by reading this book. Are you just trying to feel a bit happier about your present situation, or are you trying to improve your life to make it easier to enjoy?

Write down whatever pops into your mind – it can be a few bullet points, a long essay, or a single sentence. It could just be to pull yourself out of a bit of a rut, or it could be that you want some very specific things in life and you need to do some mindset work to achieve them.

Here's an example of a short one:

From reading this book... ... I want to learn the skills to achieve a positive outlook on life's challenges, because at the moment they seem to throw me right off course. I want to get a promotion at work within the next year, but I know I need to improve my confidence first. I want to experience something more than just my normal routine, because I'm bored and stressed and that's no longer cutting it.

You may find a specific list of goals easier:

I want to...
-Achieve a more positive outlook
-Become more confident and memorable to my bosses and colleagues
-Enrich my daily life
-Reduce my stress levels

Or perhaps a diary entry is more your style to reflect on your reasons for doing this challenge. Either way, as long as you know why you're bothering to read this book and complete its daily challenges, you can look back once you've finished and see if you think you've achieved what you wanted to, or at least have the skills and the routine to go ahead and achieve the longer term goals in the future.

Daily non-negotiables
Every day throughout this challenge, your routine should include the following:

• Write down 3 things you feel grateful for in your life. If you can only come up with one, that's completely fine, but make sure you come up with at least one. It can be the same every day, but if you can then get creative, and find new ones every time.

• Write down 3 things you've done that made someone else feel good/improved their life. It doesn't have to be that day, it can be something in the past, as long as you focus on the good you have done.

• 10 minutes of mindfulness meditation OR 20 minutes of cardio exercise.

Find a realistic time in your diary to work these things in every day, for at least the next 10 days.

If you're new to mindfulness and want some guidance, I recommend the Calm App and using the Body Scans as a place to start. Otherwise Headspace and Smiling Minds apps are also a good place to begin. Remember – I've not been paid or otherwise incentivized to make this or any other recommendation in this book. I only recommend what I truly believe works, and most of what I suggest will be what I already advise to patients on a regular basis.

For the final step before starting the 10 Day program, open a brand new document, or get a totally new page ready. Write out the following list and rate these areas of your life out of 10. 10/10 means that you're completely satisfied with the current state of that area of your life, and 0/10 means you have absolutely nothing within that category that you're happy with. You will need to be able to put this part of your prep work away and not have to look at it again until the challenge is complete.

My Ratings List

Health and wellness overall: Do you feel satisfied with how healthy you are? Do you spend your whole time worrying about health problems or how you look? Do you feel confident in your body and trust it to serve your needs?

Daily diet:
Body health:
Mental health:
Physical fitness:
Relationships overall:

Do you have satisfying, fulfilling relationships with the people in your life? Do you know you need to make more effort, or perhaps that your relationships aren't as positive as they could be? Do you have people that you can talk to, share your inner thoughts with and go to for advice?

Partner (if applicable):
Family:
Close friends:
Wider circle of acquaintances:
Daily social interactions:
Professional therapists (if applicable):
Intellectual stimulation overall: Do you feel stimulated

intellectually? Do you read for pleasure and learn new words? Do you feel like your brain is wasted on mundane tasks or are you getting the most out of your grey matter? Does your brain light up with joy and creativity every day?

Learning new things:

Using developed skills:

Having fun and laughter:

Work: Do you find your work fulfilling? Does it pay you enough? Do you enjoy talking with your colleagues or boss?

Type of work itself:

Colleagues:

Boss:

Salary:

Now that you have rated all these areas of your life, put away your ratings and don't look at them again until the end of the challenge. You've now done all the prep work and you can continue on to start the challenge.

You can either do each day completely separately, and complete just that day's challenge (alongside your non-negotiables), or you can do the challenge cumulatively, and try to complete each new challenge every day as well as all the previous challenges so far.

The 10-Day Challenge is not about being perfect, so don't worry if you forget a day – just pick up where you left off as soon as you can. If one or two of the challenges sound like your worst nightmare, then replace them with one of the other challenges for that day. This isn't about having something else to stress about and achieve – it's for giving you tools and the space to use them. The purpose of completing this series of challenges is to build your resilience against the ups and downs of life, to be able to maintain optimism even through tough times, to increase your self-esteem and to find space in your life to build relationships within your network and community. All of these things make you happier, healthier, and more able to withstand an unpredictable world and changing society.

All of these positive things are possible for you within the next ten days.

DAY 1: SPREAD THE LOVE

So presumably by this point you've spent a day or two getting prepped – you've got your daily non-negotiables written into a realistic time every day for the next 10 days, you know what your goals are and you feel pumped to rise to the 10 day challenge to get your everything on track...hell yes.

The first challenge is a gentle one to ease you into the daily extras. This starting point is about making your day a little less about you.

Today's Challenge:

Give a sincere, genuine, well thought-out compliment to at least one person, but preferably three different people. The full challenge is detailed a little further on.

So why bother?

Giving someone a compliment is the ultimate selfish act - it makes **us** happy. Doing someone a favour likewise makes **us** happy.

Why does it feel good to give to others? Well, because we are social creatures, we're hardwired to want to benefit the society we live in, and our brains reward us with a healthy dose of dopamine when we do. Sounds hard to believe sometimes, with what gets portrayed in the news every day, but it's the NORM to want to help each other out. Yes, that's right, human beings JUST WANT TO BE GOOD. Read that over again and again and it might get you through the days when it feels like every bastard is out there to get you.

But you don't have to believe me. I might be a barefoot hippy with unwashed elbows handing out flowers in a riot (My elbows are perfectly clean thank you, but that's beside the   point).
Research shows that receiving compliments makes us perform better at motor tasks. One study had participants learn a tapping sequence with their hands – those who received praise during the learning phase had better recall of the sequence later on. By complimenting someone at work, you're doing more than making them feel warm and fuzzy, you might be helping them have a more productive day – there is a catch though, as if your compliment isn't genuine it may have the opposite effect.

Giving a genuine compliment is even better for the giver – you'll be left with higher self-esteem and growing confidence. There are tons of studies in this area, and they all have similar conclusions: give good and decent praise and it'll help you out.

A man named Shawn Achor has spent years in the field of happiness research, and his studies have shown that the people who give the most praise are TEN TIMES more likely to have a productive day than their praise-stingy colleagues, and are more likely to be PROMOTED above those colleagues.

There is an ongoing, eight-decade long study into happiness, currently led by Robert Waldinger, who did an excellent TEDtalk on the subject. It has found that the greatest predictor of health and happiness in the long-term is social connection, and genuine compliments are an awesome way to build, strengthen, and deepen social connections. Three-quarters of a century of research has shown that "high quality, stable relationships" are the BEST predictor of staying alive beyond middle age, and feeling happy about it. Cholesterol levels, blood pressure and other key health indicators were less important than social connection. Incredible really.

So if you want to live a long, healthy, happy life, full of strong bonds and deep friendships, where you have high self-esteem, earn more money and receive more respect, you should start by making somebody else's day.

This day's challenge comes in a couple of parts. Firstly, choose your guinea pigs.

You'll need at least one of the following:

Guinea pig 1: a close friend or relative that you know very well

Guinea pig 2: a work colleague

Guinea pig 3: an acquaintance.

Our close friend or relative guinea pig is the first. For some people, this will be the easiest one, and for others, the most daunting. Doesn't matter either way, just get it done. As long as you compliment at least one of the following guinea pigs, you can call it a day if you so desire. If you want to start with a bang, try all three in one day…you'll feel amazing afterwards.

Guinea pig 1: Close friend/relative

First off, think about something you admire about them. This will only work if it's genuine, so put a little effort into coming up with a sincere compliment.

I'll use my sister as my example, which is a bit of a cheat because I find it very easy to admire her. A few years before I started writing my book, she had a major horseriding accident that required extensive, multiple surgeries on her leg, and has left her unable to walk properly, possibly forever. She was lucky not to need amputation after smashing up her lower leg and foot to the point where they lost count after adding up the first 18 breaks and fractures.

But what does my sister's limp have to do with

anything? Well, she's a vibrant, active 30-something who rides her horse every day and is chairwoman of the riding club for the entire district. She's a successful professional, has a beautiful marriage and family, and is busy all the time. And she hasn't let this stop her one tiny modicum of a bit. It took her 11 months, but she got back on her horse after being told she wouldn't ride again. She's finding ways to exercise that her now limited ankle movement allows for. She may have the occasional complaint on the more painful days, but she ALWAYS punctures it with what she's grateful for and how far she's come. So I found it easy to step up and tell her that I think she's a badass. A total badass.

It doesn't have to be that epic. You might just send your good friend a text asking her for some advice on a colour scheme because you know she has such a good eye for that kind of thing. You might tell your dad that you had a win at work today, and you think it must be his genes because he's always been your inspiration for that kind of thing. Phone your mum, tell her she's awesome at something you know she's awesome at. Make your compliment count.

Guinea pig 2: colleague/professional acquaintance

The work colleague. Whether you're self-employed, work alone at home or sit in a cubicle surrounded by thousands of other identical cubicles, there will be someone with whom you come into professional contact that you can wing a compliment towards.

To avoid awkwardness or misunderstandings, make the compliment to do with personality, work ethic, recent completion of project etc, and sidestep compliments about physical characteristics, as this could be misconstrued as a flirtation (or general creepiness!) Compliments about physical appearance can be easier to dismiss as non-genuine as well.

You can also take the focus of your praise away from

the compliment itself, by adding context, to help the other person accept the compliment as true and genuine. So rather than saying "your presentation was really good today", try saying "your presentation was really good today, were you nervous beforehand?"

Or "that idea you came up with in the meeting was brilliant, have you been thinking on it for a while?" Or "you always send everything to me on time, that makes my job much easier so thanks." You get the idea.

Guinea pig 3: someone you don't know that well. Finally, the acquaintance. How many times do you scroll down your newsfeed, hit 'like' and then continue scrolling? It's an easy way to show someone you think their photo or words are cool, but without actually putting in any effort. Next time, try "that looks beautiful, where are you?" or "so happy for you getting married, congratulations, you look so right together" or "argh your cat is so cute".

Just try it. You'll feel good. You might reconnect with a friend you've lost touch with, or never knew that well in the first place. You might be surprised at the results.

If the newsfeed isn't your thing, try it in the real world (gasp!) on a barista, a local dog walker, or the cashier. A casual compliment about someone's glasses, adorable pet, or topnotch latte-making skills can go a long way.

DAY 2: CONNECT WITH A FRIEND YOU LOVE

The first day's challenge should have made you feel good, made a few other people feel good, and made you more promotable, more likeable, and better equipped to understand who in your life may be the best person to go to for differing things. Write down what you achieved yesterday if you haven't already, or it'll be too easy to forget how hard you've worked when you come to reflect on what you've achieved in these ten days. It's super important to be reminded of the hard work we've put in once the challenge is over. Day 2 takes us somewhere pretty comfortable, hopefully.

Today's Challenge:
Pick a friend or family member that you feel close to, most preferably someone who is generally supportive of you. Then pick up the phone and call them. Throughout your call, tell them about the happiness challenge you're doing, and tell them how it's going. Arrange to meet up with them in person if possible (it doesn't have to be today), put it in the diary, and stick to it. A video call counts as an in-person meeting in times of need. So why bother?

It's no great secret that spending time with friends and loved ones can bring us a sense of belonging and contentment, but have you ever stopped to wonder if the benefits are quantifiable? The world's longest study into happiness has managed not only to quantify the benefits, but track them in the same set of people for more than seventy-five years, as mentioned in the previous chapter.

That's right, through what the current director Robert Waldinger terms as "luck and persistence", generations of researchers have undertaken to continue the study that began with a cohort of teenagers who are now in their eighties and beyond, and whose children and grandchildren are now participating. Through regular blood tests, brain scans, body scans, surveys, questionnaires, interviews and observations, these researchers discovered one key component to what makes a happy, healthy life: relationships. Good ones, specifically.

The researchers decided to go back through decades and decades of data to see if there was a common pattern to who lived a long, happy life, and who didn't. The answer was surprising.

The key predictor for living to well past the average age expectancy was not cholesterol or blood pressure – it was stable, high quality relationships. Those who were in a happy, supportive, committed relationship in middle age were much more likely to be protected from brain degradation, to make it to old age, and to be happy about it. The same could be said for those who had close social ties with family and friends, and rarely reported loneliness.

In one sentence: close social ties make you healthy, happy, and less likely to get dementia.

Given that one in five adult Americans report feeling lonely at any given time, and that the UK is the loneliness capital of Europe, this could have a huge impact on public health care. It is important to remember that just having a partner doesn't equate to happiness, as people can feel lonely in a marriage or a crowd of friends, but it is rather having a partner and network that you feel are supportive and can be relied upon, who make you feel safe, secure and loved.

Another set of research highlighted the number of interactions with strong ties (family, friends, colleagues) and weak ties (casual acquaintances, cashiers, neighbours you recognise) and their effect upon happiness levels. This study found that a greater number of interactions with strong ties was linked to a greater sense of happiness, as expected. Somewhat unexpectedly, this was also true of weak ties, but only when someone is new to a community. Therefore, a sense of belonging needs to be established to contribute to happiness, but after that the stronger ties play a bigger role in happiness levels. When new to a community, happiness can be increased by simple interactions such as smiling at people on the street, but once that sense of belonging is established, happiness increases more with deeper, more personal interactions.

So there we have it, loving relationships and strong community networks protect your body, your brain, and create happiness. Today's challenge comes as a variety of options. The most preferable option is the one laid out at the beginning of the chapter, which involves the strengthening of a close bond that already exists. But if this isn't your first time doing the 10-day challenge, you've recently moved house, or for some reason nobody is available for a chat today, I've written out a few others that count as completing today's challenge.

Other options for today's challenge include the following.

If you're new to an area:

- Research and join a community project, sports team, book club or art society, whatever floats your boat. Virtual exercise classes can count in a pinch.
- Start a conversation with 2 new people today, whether that be a local dogwalker or a cashier

at the local shop – you never know where those conversations may take you. You only have to comment on the weather and tell them you're new to the area for the conversation to count! If social distancing is currently occurring, take it online if you can't get a chat with a loved one.

- Comment on a local forum or group or start a community project. Maybe even just wave at a neighbour.

Whether you're new or established:
- Start a new hobby that takes you into contact with other people, whether it be knitting or rock-climbing – nothing creates strong ties and close friendships more quickly than having a shared passion.
- Join a social media group dedicated to a particular hobby that you're interested in. Try to find one that has a supportive, friendly atmosphere.
- Volunteer at an old people's home visiting or calling those who need some company – extra happiness comes from charitable acts and someone else gets to feel a little less lonely too. Perhaps you could even volunteer to video chat to someone if the care home can set it up.
- Set a regular weekly or monthly date to hang out with some friends, ie agree on the first Friday of every month for dinner and a film, or for a group video call.
- Instead of sitting on the couch mindlessly watching television with your partner, actively do something together, whether that be gardening, playing scrabble, taking up that new hobby together or just having a simple a walk around the block.

Loneliness is a complex issue with far-reaching psychological and physiological consequences. If you are really struggling with loneliness and are concerned about your mental or physical wellbeing, and feel that the challenges in day 2 are beyond you for now, you should seek the advice of your health professional.

DAY 3: YOUR WORLD CAN BE A BETTER PLACE

The first two challenges have been all about connecting with others, and you should now be compiling quite a list of people with whom you've had a meaningful dialogue so far on your challenge. Today's challenge is partly about further increasing our connection to the other people that form our society, and making us feel good about our role within that society.

Multiple studies have confirmed that donating to charity is an easy way to feel good about yourself. Whether through monetary gifts, volunteering or dropping off supplies, our individual actions make a difference every single day. After all, what's the point of being the richest human in the universe if you feel horrible about the world? If you wake up every day in your expensive sheets in your expensive house with an expensive view, and still feel sour about life?

The happiest people in the world are community-centred individuals.

Today's challenge:
- Research and choose a charity or cause that aligns with your beliefs
- Donate either your time, your money or some products they're in need of.

You can choose a huge global organization, or stay more local. Really think about what matters to you, and where you'd like to see yourself having a positive impact.

So why bother?

This one is super simple. Spend some money on helping other people or a cause you feel warm and fuzzy about, and you'll compound the goodness around the world. Studies since the 1970's have shown that happy people like themselves, and feel hope for the future. A good way to get both of these birds down with a single pebble is to donate to a charity in some way, and so build yourself some resilience through self-esteem and optimism. When you receive updates or are involved with a cause you believe in, you see the difference being made, the plans for the future being laid down, and the ways in which you can directly have an effect. There are lots of ways you can "make a difference" to the world, some of which don't necessarily involve spending your money, and here are just a few examples:

- Pick a charitable cause that you believe in, research a charity where you know the money will actually go to the cause you want to help, and set up a monthly direct debit. Try to pick one where you get an update on a regular basis that informs you of the good you have helped to promote.
- An easy way to donate to a charity that spends their money wisely is through The Life You Can Save, or Change Path. These are not-for-profits who have dedicated themselves to researching the charities where you get the best bang for your buck in terms of the money going to the cause instead of advertising or executive salaries.
- Have a look at a crowdfunding campaign website to see if there's a product or business on there

that you can get behind. You'll have the pleasure of knowing you helped a startup succeed, whilst making the world a better place. Depending on the size of your donation, you may sometimes get a thank you note, stake in the company, or first test of the product.

- See if there's a local pet shelter that needs your old towels or sheets. You get a bonus of clearing out some space, and knowing that something cute and fuzzy is a little warmer thanks to you.

- Search out your local foodbank, find out what they need most and get in the habit of buying an extra tin or two every time you shop.

- Join a local litter clean-up project. This is a bonus way to meet fellow like-minded people too.

- Have a look at the free ways you can make the word a better place. I downloaded the Ecosia search engine, where searches translate into the rebuilding of forests. They have fun infographics they release each month to show you exactly how and where their projects are taking effect.

These examples are just the best I could come up with, and represent only a tiny fraction of a drop of the human kindness going on across the world. If you have a great tip on contributing to society that you'd like to share, message The Happiness Wagon through social media or the contact form on thehappinesswagon.com, and I may share your story with my readers.

Given the way the world can feel like a merry-go-round of disasters with the current news cycle and clickbait-y headlines, donating to charity isn't just about trying to make a change. It's also about exerting control over what can feel like an overwhelming mess, if we don't take steps to filter the information we receive, and to make positive action with the news we are exposed to on a regular basis.

As humans, we feel happier when we have some sense

of control in events as they unfold. If you find yourself reading news articles and feeling hopeless, these are the causes you should look into supporting. Feeling terrible about the state of the world and doing nothing whatsoever about it will simply cause you to feel more depressed.

Consider your regular donation of money or time, or other contributions, as a "happiness buffer" against the news. You CAN make a difference, and when you know deep down that your contributions are helping someone or something that you believe in, you can wake up every day and feel great about the future of our society. That feeling of hope and control is the foundation of resilience.

N.B. Please only donate money if you can afford it – if you're in dire financial straits, there are plenty of excellent resources available to help you out. Start with the Barefoot Investor by Scott Pape (with whom I have no affiliation of any kind).

DAY 4: SUSTAINABLE HAPPINESS

Want to feel like you earn several thousand dollars more per year, are part of something bigger than yourself, increase your sense of community and do all this with very little effort? Time to start recycling.

Today's Challenge:
Put in place at least one actionable change that will make your ecological impact slightly more positive.

So why bother?
If the footage of dying whale babies and their grieving mothers hasn't been enough to motivate you towards mindful consumerism, then you can have a look at the totally selfish reasons to say no to that straw.

Sustainable, eco-friendly behaviours are closely linked with happiness and satisfaction with life. Contrary to the widely-held belief that environmental sustainability comes at the price of individual freedom, people who adopt behaviours that promote environmental conservation are much more likely to report higher levels of satisfaction with life and increased sense of community. Perhaps there's an element of truth to that stereotype of the smug New Earth dude wearing hemp trousers and espousing the benefits of his bicycle, but don't let that put you off.

The link is now so established that it has its own phrase. "Sustainable happiness" was a term coined by Catherine O'Brien, professor at Cape Breton University, Canada. The phrase refers to happiness that contributes to individual, community and global wellbeing, without the exploitation of other people, the environment, or future generations.

Through millions of responses to surveys like the World Values Survey, the Gallup World Poll and the European Social Survey, it has been found that the happier people are those that recycle, limit waste, and reduce their carbon footprint where they can. People who agreed with the statement "it is important to care for the environment" were found to have an increase in happiness by 0.2, compared to those who strongly disagreed with the statement.

0.2 sounds pretty pathetic, right? Not when you consider that this increase in happiness is the same as when increasing self-rated wealth from "low income" to "middle income". That's **the equivalent to several thousand dollars per year**. It's the equivalent to reaching the peak on the income-happiness scale.

Consumer culture encourages the constant creation of waste, which is already known to have negative consequences for the environment. But this is also having psychological consequences at the individual and societal level whereby we are making ourselves miserable.

The correlation between actions to reduce waste and an increase in happiness have been shown in the Zero Waste Project in Denmark, The Happiness Initiative Sustainable Seattle, and many more. Although correlation and causation do not mean the same thing, the groundwork for future studies has been laid.

The Happiness Research Institute theorises as to some

of the possibilities behind the correlation between happiness and sustainability:

- *Happier people are more likely to care about the environment and therefore engage in sustainable behaviours*

- *Sustainable behaviours directly cause happiness Sustainable behaviours cause an increase in feelings of civil society, trust and participation in community.*

These theories may be all wrong or may work in combination. It could be that happiness is increased by the added feelings of control and autonomy from taking charge of household waste production, given that these feelings are strongly related to happiness, as you'll find out in the next chapter.

Regardless of the reasons why, the bare fact is that happy people often engage in sustainable behaviours. Today's challenge details: engage in three extra sustainable behaviours that you haven't previously tried:

- If you don't already have one, get a recycling bin and use it. I just use a cardboard box that has seen better days, and replace it occasionally once it looks too limp to continue. Make sure you know what counts as recyclable before chucking anything in there.

- Compost your waste food. Did you know a single lettuce can take more than twenty-five years to decompose in landfill? Food in landfill essentially becomes embalmed in plastic and waste, and as a result releases noxious gases for a long time while it gradually breaks down.

- Replace single-use plastic items with reusable versions – buy a reusable takeaway coffee cup, get reusable food wraps instead of plastic clingfilm or sandwich bags, take a refillable water bottle with you instead of buying plastic bottles out.

- Sign a petition to stop supermarkets wrapping fruit and vegetables in plastic, and in the meantime, buy only loose vegetables or use paper bags.

- Have meat-free days every week. On any day that you avoid meat, your personal carbon footprint for that day is

roughly   halved.
 - Bring your own bags to the supermarket. My best tip for remembering your own shopping bags is to get a foldable one to keep in your workbag, so any last-minute nipping to the shop doesn't have to cost you the earth.   - Get biodegradable binbags to replace the ones that never biodegrade.
 - Research the feasibility of adding solar power to your house   or   business.
 - Go electric. Next time you buy a car, consider the wide range of e-vehicles out there. It won't be long before that's a legal requirement in most countries anyway, and you can be one of the early adopters of a form of transport that doesn't literally poison the air as you move.

I now use my own water bottle, invested in a KeepCup, go meat-free at least four days a week, take my own shopping bags with me everywhere, and I'm starting to replace kitchen essentials such as clingfilm and plastic Tupperware with more sustainable alternatives. My bathroom has been ninety per-cent plastic-free for over a year now.

The possibilities are endless.

DAY 5: MAKE YOUR WORK MEANINGFUL

This doesn't necessarily mean you have to change jobs or give up all your possessions to work as a volunteer in a soup kitchen. It's possible to do all that of course, but you can look for ways to make your current work have more meaning.

Today's Challenge:

Two or three actions that make your work feel more purpose-driven, meaningful and positive.

Why bother?

The seven happiest jobs in the UK were found in 2016 to range from an annual salary of £18k to £70k, as a gardener and medical practitioner respectively. Others on the list included engineer, nurse, teacher, personal assistant, and construction worker. Personally, I think what that list shows is that beyond your basic needs, what you earn doesn't matter one iota. The research backs this up.

In 2016, it was reported that 20-35 year olds globally were more likely than ever to start their own businesses, and be more successful at it than baby boomers. It's possible that in the era of the millennial millionaire, the idea of working for someone else looks less enticing, but also possible that more millennials than ever before are looking for meaning from their work.

According to studies by The Happiness Research Institute, we care more about our purpose than we do about our salary, by a long shot. The more motivated you feel, the more likely you have a greater sense of purpose at work, and so the happier you'll be.

Before we get on to the challenge for today, find out if you're motivated at work and ask yourself the following in line with the Job Satisfaction Index:

1. Do I feel proud of my job?
2. Do I experience personal satisfaction from my job?
3. Do I experience making work-related progress?
4. Do I experience my job as meaningful?
5. Do I feel like I develop my competencies?

If you answered "yes" to most of or all those questions, happy days! You are motivated at work and likely feel like your job has a sense of purpose. Go and say thank you to your boss or your employees and wallow in the extra joy gratitude brings.

If you answered "no" to most or all of those five questions, you may want to consider a proactive approach to increasing your motivation at work. Research has shown repeatedly that the most important factors for job satisfaction are purpose, mastery and work-life balance. If we identify the meaning and purpose behind our work, and understand the necessity of our role to achieve those ends this makes us feel more satisfied by the work we do. If we feel competent and have the opportunity to develop our skills further, we get to feel good about our day job. And if we can balance out time spent at work with time spent on leisure, family and enjoyment, we feel good about it.

Other factors for happiness at work include the people in charge, achievements, our colleagues, autonomy and salary. Salary is actually the least important indicator for happiness out of all of these, and once we can get out basic needs covered, we generally find it more important to earn more than those around us than to earn more overall.

Purpose and meaning are so important that it has been found that workers in smaller companies are much happier than those at larger corporations. This could be because it's incredibly obvious what you contribute in a smaller workforce, and precisely the impact you personally create is much easier to see and measure, when you only have a handful of colleagues.

Today's challenge details: to increase your sense of purpose and job satisfaction, pick 2-3 options from below.

For employees:

- Ask your boss specifically what the company's goals are for this month, and how you could be better contributing towards them.

- Ask your boss for a review for some constructive feedback – where your competencies are and where you could work to improve. Strengthening your confidence in your own qualities and competencies helps you become a happier, more motivated worker.

- Discuss work stress with those higher up the chain – companies that do this have happier, more productive workers

- Develop your skills, and deepen them in a specific area by spending time on training, professional events and buddying up with someone who can do it well already. This will increase your mastery, thereby increasing your happiness, and your value to your company or your clients.

For leaders:
- Make the company goals clear.
- Give constructive, simple and fast feedback to workers on how they are achieving these goals.
- Tell individual employees why their work is important, even on seemingly trivial tasks. If employees know how they are contributing to the company, they feel a real purpose to their work.
- If you're the only employee of you one-person band, figure out which jobs you do most regularly, and write down the ways in which those jobs help you towards your business goals. Especially for tasks you find boring, this will help you motivate yourself when you're feeling a bit exasperated.
- Donate as a company – money, time or skills! Good publicity is never to be sniffed at, but charitable donation also gives you and your employees a greater sense of upward purpose.
- Hold meetings where leaders and workers discuss things together. This increases trust in management which helps increase employee satisfaction, and you may be surprised by how much more your workers are capable of.
- Make space for workers to discuss work-life balance with you. If employees feel stressed, overworked, inadequate or frustrated, you should know about it, and you should help find solutions. Companies where this discussion takes place have much happier workers, higher employee retention, and better turnover.

The above can all apply to anyone with whom you come into regular professional contact.

If you yourself are running a small business, or even a

one (wo)man show, it can be bloody hard to find the mythical work-life balance. Consider taking on an employee or contractor, or even a business partner, to share the load and enable you to have a breather here and there. If that's not doable, try to find a buddy who understands the situation and can act as a bit of a sounding board. Business forums can be a good place to start online if you don't have anyone you can think of in your existing network.

If you absolutely hate your job, your boss is an a-hole and there's no way in hell you ever want to help the company achieve anything ever, consider the effect that's going to be having on your brain. Fight or flight will abound, anger and resentment will be brewing, and dare I say it – you're quite likely to be taking out your frustration on the people who don't deserve it, whether that's other employees at the company or your baffled loved ones. Personal growth, relationship strengthening, income growing and contentment are all infinitely harder to achieve if you're spending 80% of your waking life miserable. If you have no option to increase your happiness in your current job, either it's time to make some drastic changes to your work situation, or to pour time and effort into maximising the joy you get from your leisure time.

If you're struggling with your career, talk to a licensed psychologist or career counsellor to get some professional help in improving your situation.

DAY 6: MAKING SADNESS YOUR SUCCESS

Negative emotions are the ones that make us feel sad, upset, angry or hateful. Left unchecked, they can have disproportionately negative consequences on a person's life, but when dealt with appropriately, they actually make us happier, healthier, better at coping and less stressed.

Today's Challenge:

To acknowledge, label and reframe a negative thought process.

So why bother?

When we don't acknowledge what we're feeling and try to suppress it, because we think that will make us feel better, our subconscious continues to dwell on the negative and may result in harmful behaviours:

A 2010 study found that people were more likely to overeat when they suppressed thoughts about food instead of acknowledging them, particularly when attempting to lose weight.

A 2011 study found that trying to suppress a thought before going to sleep meant that participants had an increased number of dreams associated with it.

A 2013 study of people with history of exposure to traumatic events and substance abuse found that suppression of unwanted thoughts led to increased likelihood of suffering from post-traumatic stress disorder and addiction. The best predictor of both PTSD and addiction was NOT the length or intensity of the trauma but the amount of thought suppression the individual engaged in, whilst mindfulness made people less likely to suffer both PTSD and addiction.

Another 2013 study found that negative thought suppression five minutes before going to sleep causes increased number of nightmares.

Over the years, what these and many more studies have shown are the harmful effects of thought suppression, from merely dreaming more of the unwanted topic or having nightmares, to post-traumatic stress disorder and to the self-harming behaviours of overeating and addiction. Negative emotions provide indicators to what is going on around us, and are useful warning signs of financial, health or relationship woes that may prompt us to change our behaviours for the better.

So what should I do?

Acknowledge your emotions – the more powerful the acknowledgement, the greater the effect. So just telling yourself "I feel upset" is a good start, writing it down is even better, and telling someone else that you trust could be best, whether that be a friend or a therapist.

Understand which emotion you are feeling without trying to change it – try and give the emotion a name, such as anger, sadness, frustration, hopelessness, exhaustion, disappointment…if you can't name it then make up your own.

Practice mindfulness to enable yourself to cope better when faced with negative emotions. There are many apps that can help with this, such as Calm and Headspace (I have no affiliation with either, but regularly recommend them to my patients).

If you are experiencing suicidal thoughts, depression or other mental health difficulties, seek advice from a qualified counsellor, therapist or your doctor – just like many other types of medical issues, there are some things we cannot fix all by ourselves.

Today's challenge details: Write down three sentences throughout today, where each sentence:

-Labels a negative emotion you may be feeling and -Explains what that feeling relates to and

-Qualifies the negative with a statement that begins with "but"

-Reframes the process to focus on something positive that has/can come from it.

Psychologist Jonathan Adler found that experiencing a mix of emotions has a positive effective on mental well-being for several weeks afterwards. Whilst acknowledging the negative, also try to follow it with the word "but" and a hint of positivity, like "I feel sad that this situation is happening **but** I know I can figure it out **and I feel cheerful** that I'm at least trying to resolve it". Or "I'm angry that my partner forgot to make the bed, **but** I know there were no bad intentions, **and I'm glad** I was able to communicate that I was annoyed in a calm way".

DAY 7: HOBBIES AND RELATIONSHIPS

It's important that life doesn't just revolve around work and survival. For decades, studies have shown that the building blocks of happiness include time for creativity and fun. When our basic needs of safety, food and shelter are met, we can start to look around us for ways in which we can explore our own strengths and weaknesses, and enjoy doing so.

Today's challenge: Take an interest in something you've never bothered with before. If you have a loved one who has been trying to get you into their hobby for a while, give it a go as this can double as a good way to build relationships. Otherwise, just try and invest your time in something that brings you joy, not added stress. Examples of some activities:

- Drawing (if you don't know how to draw, I would recommend "Drawing on the Right Side of the Brain" by Betty Edwards)
- Education – as a bonus, there are lots of free online courses available at edx, coursera, teachable and other such websites.

- Gardening
- Knitting
- Making your own soap, shampoo, face masks, moisturiser and other skin care
- Musical instrument
- Painting
- Woodworking

That's a very short list of the top of my head, and is barely even the tip of the iceberg of what's available. You can double up the social aspect by jumping on a video chat with a loved one and learning together.

So why bother?

Hobbies that give you an end product continue to give you joy in several ways – from the learning and creative process to the outcome that you can enjoy and share with other people, whether that's playing them their favourite song on the guitar or handing them a new scarf. For example, gardeners get a dopamine rush just from harvesting the fruits of their labours (pun intended), and that's before they've taken photos and posted to social media or gardening groups. Gardeners likely experience a high when they harvest their produce as a result of several hundred thousand years of "hunter-gatherer" behaviour, which trained us to seek out nourishing food. This dopamine rush is exploited by retail outlets, as the experience of shopping is similar to foraging and finding success – which is why gardening may also protect you from the urge to spend money to cheer yourself up.

Hobbies have been found to increase happiness across knitters, crafters, sportspeople and more, from childhood to later life. It seems that sport is more of an indicator for happiness in children and early adulthood, and that hobbies become more important as you age. Hobbies are not only important for happiness, but also for challenging and protecting your brain from common problems associated with ageing.

One study found that extroverts tend to be happier as a result of engaging in sporting activity, whilst introverts gained more from self-directed hobbies. But don't worry too much about trying to scientifically match your age and personality to the hobby that best suits you – just try a few out and see what works.

DAY 8: GET YOUR BLOOD PUMPING

Congratulations! You've arrived at the point where you get to raise a sweat. This one is about you, and love it or hate it, you're going to have to step up your steps to step up your happiness.

The Challenge:

Exercise for 20 minutes extra. This can be all at once, or by adding a few minutes of exercise several times throughout the day. Today is the day where you add a little cardio into your life. At lunchtime if possible, but do whatever works for you around your schedule. Think you're too busy to exercise? Well, guess again – there are some very smart people who have found you don't actually have to exercise for very long at all each day to get some awesome results, physically and mentally. And you can even break it down into 5 minute blocks if you like.

Current guidelines for exercise tend to revolve around the 150 minutes a week that have been recommended for the last two decades. However, you don't need to do as much exercise as you think to be happier and healthier – plenty of research now shows how most of the benefits of exercise can be gleaned in 20 minutes, either all at once or cumulatively through the day. More and more research is

coming out that says you don't have to do much at all, as long as you do some regularly.
So why bother?

If you're an employee, there may even be a chance that your boss will let you have an extra long lunch break to give you time to exercise, at least a few times a week.

And why would your boss come over so generous? Well, you can show them the research proving that employees who get physical at lunchtime are **much more productive** for the rest of the afternoon than their lazier colleagues. A Leeds Metropoltian University Study found that individual workers also outshone their own performance on days when they exercised at lunchtime, compared to days when they didn't. Not only did people report better time management, higher productivity, and more positive professional relationships on days when they made it to the gym, but they reported higher satisfaction levels at the end of the working day.

It's a no-brainer - if you're a boss, get working on providing your workforce with a gym membership and/or extra time allowance for exercising – you'll likely retain more workers and get way more out of your team. So, what's in it for me? If the above hasn't been enough to convince you to at least take the stairs, there's not much chance the rest of this chapter will persuade you…but it's always worth a shot.

Endorphins get released during exercise. -These molecules of happiness help counteract feelings of stress, can make you feel high, and may be responsible for a large number of the benefits of exercise.

You'll sleep better when you exercise regularly. -Better quality sleep has been shown in various studies to aid concentration, memory and health, while making you appear more attractive and feel less stressed, even at just 10 minutes per day, with benefits maxing out at 150 minutes of exercise a week.

You'll behave better. -A study of bosses found that

those leaders who were regularly physically active had happier employees, who were less likely to report feeling victimised at work. Those bosses who were physically inactive were likely to feel more stressed and take it out on their unsuspecting employees. Exercise regularly, and become a nicer person to be around. Hooray for everybody!

You'll get excited. -When you regularly break a sweat, you'll feel more excited and enthusiastic about life. One study found that of 190 college students, those who exercised were more optimistic about life. The study also found that any day where participants exercised at a slightly higher intensity than usual, caused an even greater boost to mood for that day.

You'll have more satisfying sex (disclaimer: up to a point). Light and moderate intensity workout routines have been associated with a higher sex drive in both men and women. Although, due to the hormone testosterone, these effects go into the negative at high intensity training. Men who train excessively heavily can expect a reduced libido, while women can suffer the same along with the (usually temporary) loss or disruption of their menstrual cycle. Unless you're planning to use your lunch break to train for an iron man, however, I wouldn't worry too much.

You'll be less likely to die from anything. All-cause mortality has been found to be significantly reduced in anyone who exercises regularly, even those who exercise less than the recommended amount of 150 minutes per week of moderate intensity, or 75 minutes per week of intense exercise across 3 sessions. Research has found that people who exercised regularly at less than the recommended amount, compared with those who do no regular exercise, were 30% less likely to die from any reason, while those meeting the guidelines were 35% less likely to die from any reason. Plenty of other studies have also shown similar inverse associations with higher fitness and lower mortality.

So, here are your options for the daily challenge, should you happen to prefer a life where you're alive, happier, more well-liked, more promotable, get more beauty sleep and potentially have better sex:

- A gym class in your lunch break that gets your sweat on. Virtual bootcamps and online personal training mean that it's never been easier to workout without having to leave the house
- Stand on one leg while brushing your teeth to work out your balancing skills
- A twenty-minute power walk instead of staying at your desk in your down-time
- Two lots of ten-minute power walks - park a few streets further away, get off your bus a stop early, walk the long way around. Make space to find an extra 600 seconds for your commute
- Park further away from shops, work or home. Remember, exercise can be cumulative, so a brisk walking pace for an extra 2 minutes here and there might be the boost that gets you up to your 20 minutes
- Take the stairs instead of the escalator for the same reason
- If you're anybody's boss, do all your employees a favour and hit the exercise mat.

It doesn't really matter what you do...as long as you do it. If you haven't exercised for a while, it may be a good idea just to do a little extra walking before building up to doing anything involving weights. Where possible, if you want to go a little more hardcore, make sure you start off with supervision by a personal trainer or exercise physiologist to avoid getting injured.

DAY 9: REALISTIC OPTIMISM

Today is about understanding your frame of mind. Anyone who has made it this far and completed the challenges is already well on the way to reframing their mindset. If that includes you, then you've upped your game in your relationships, how your colleagues view you, how you use your work day and how you speak to yourself. You may have already been doing some of these things quite naturally, you may have come from a place where you're starting from scratch on creating a foundation for happiness within your mindset.

Today's challenge:

Use your gratitudes to develop your optimism. Read them and share some of them with someone else. Go over your positive impacts and actively praise yourself for every single time you have positively added to someone else's day.

So why bother?

The point of all these challenges, not just today's one, is to make your natural baseline one of realistic optimism. People with greater realistic optimism…

• Have healthier hearts: people in the highest quartile of optimism scores are the most likely to have ideal or near-ideal arterial health.

• Live longer: Optimists are more likely to take care of their bodies, recover faster from operations and get health check-ups when they need them.

• Are more successful at school and university: realistic optimists know they need to study to achieve good grades, and are more likely to feel they will be rewarded for studying, therefore they work harder than unrealistic optimists and pessimists alike, and get better grades. Children who are praised for natural intelligence over effort are more likely to choose the easiest path for fear of losing their "intelligent" status, whereas children who are praised for effort are more likely to treat challenges as learning opportunities.

• Have longer, happier marriages: optimists are no more likely to marry another optimist than anyone else, but that doesn't matter, as both partners are likely to report greater satisfaction in the relationship when one of them is an optimist.

• Earn more money: employees who are optimists are more likely to involve themselves in group activities, get along well with their coworkers and ask for a pay rise when the time is right, and so earn on average a yearly $4000 AUD more than pessimists.

• Find re-employment more quickly than pessimists: optimists tend to give themselves more options than pessimists. This means that when something bad happens, for instance being made redundant, an optimist will treat it more like an opportunity and feel more motivated to start looking for work an average of 4-6 weeks sooner than a pessimist.

As if these reasons weren't enough, there are many more studies that show optimists are happier, more popular and more satisfied with life in general than pessimists.

This is all well and good, but isn't optimism an

innate trait, where some people are just born with it?
Absolutely not! Optimism is taught and learned, just like pessimism. Children who are raised by optimists are more likely to become optimists themselves, regardless of whether the role models are their biological parents.

How can I learn optimism?

Through everything we've done so far in this 10-day challenge, you've been flexing your muscles of optimism, but today we can develop that further.

You should have been writing your three gratitudes every day already. Today, tell your gratitudes to someone too. You can even put it up on social media if that's your style – that way, other people get to see something positive as well. Read over all the gratitudes and positive actions you've written down so far, and bathe in the glory of all the things there are to enjoy in your life. Gratitude and optimism go hand in hand – think of it as a reminder to your brain that you are capable and well-adapted to the world around you. With that repetition, it becomes automatic for your brain to look for the positive spin on challenges.

With that in mind, put a positive spin on a recent difficult situation and write it down. Think of a time when you had a crap day. Your bag strap broke, you got lost on a journey, your boss yelled at you or you had an argument with a loved one. Think about something that happened as a result that wasn't terrible – perhaps someone went out of their way to help you, you had a bit of an adventure, or you colleagues commiserated with you, or you learned something about a relationship that could help you better communicate with each other in the future. Optimists see problems as opportunities, not insurmountable obstacles, and as a result they overcome those problems, and feel secure in themselves that they will continue to do so, no matter what life throws at them.

Praise yourself for effort, and not for intelligence or

results – realistic optimists achieve more because they subconsciously feel that they will be rewarded for working hard. If you have worked hard for something, think about how wonderful it is to have done your best, no matter what the result.

If you find yourself complaining about something today, use the optimist's trick of the final sentence on your complaint. It may look something like this:

"There was such a huge queue at the bank today, I didn't get time to eat my lunch. BUT now I know for next time, I will just bring my food with me if I want to do a job like that at lunchtime again"

"They've raised prices at my favourite coffee shop again. BUT that probably means they must be keeping the quality high, and that's why I like their coffee in the first place"

"My colleagues have left me to do all the work again. BUT I know I can do a great job and show my boss how valuable I am, and next time I can put my name on it from the start so I get the credit due to me".

It's fairly simple, and we covered some of this on day 6. If you listen to some positive people when they speak, you'll notice most optimists do it. Use the last sentence to conclude something positive or something that you learned which you can go forward and use in the future.

Fill your life with positivity. If you're active on social media, start following pages that promote things that make you feel happy. Good news pages are a good start, but also think about things you really enjoy reading about, whether that's car maintenance or vegetable growing or cooking tips. **Talk often to your friends** who are positive - try to really listen to how they speak about their own problems.

Remember, realistic optimism is grounded in reality. It doesn't mean that you ignore what's really going on around you, and just pretend everything is fine when it isn't. If the kitchen is on fire, you don't sit at the table drinking your tea – you get up and move, quickly, and take steps to put it out and make yourself safe, or you might call in the professionals to help. Realistic optimists get the fire put out, acknowledge their sadness about the loss of their favourite placemats, and then they get excited about the opportunity to redecorate.

Allow yourself to feel negative emotions. Don't try to ignore them or block them out – if something is making you feel sad, angry, or hurt, try to understand why you are feeling what you're feeling, and if it is within your control to change it, create a plan to make those changes. If it's outside of your control, feel your emotions, acknowledge them, and share them with someone you trust.

"Positive vibes only" as a movement has great intentions, but it simply **isn't a realistic expectation** from life. If you attempt to block out sadness, you will take out a range of emotions with it, including genuine happiness. Remove the pressure to **only** feel happy vibes, and suddenly it becomes a lot easier to enjoy them.

Understand that happiness is not an end destination – it is a skill that you learn that makes the journey easier. A job promotion is not the key to bring you happiness, but happiness may bring you a job promotion.

DAY 10: MEASURE YOUR OUTCOMES

You've nearly made it! The last day of the 10 Day Challenge has arrived. Today is pick-your-own, so you get to decide.

Today's Challenge:
Pick your favourite two challenges to repeat them
AND
Decide which way to go now.

As well as writing your gratitudes, your positive impact on other people, and getting your exercise or mindfulness today, you should now have a few go-to options for building into your everyday life. Repeat the challenges that you want to, whether it's the ones you found the easiest, or the ones you found the most challenging.

Going on from here, you may want to redo the challenge from start to finish on repeat for 90 days. You may just want to continue with the daily non-negotiables, or just one of them every day on rotation. Whatever you decide to do to from here, diarise it. If it's in your calendar, you're much more likely to do it. Now that you've finished your challenge, head back to the Preparation chapter and repeat the ratings list of various aspects of your life that you did before you started. **Don't peek** at your first one until after you've done it again, you want to be able to compare without cheating.

Now compare the ratings list in front of you with the one you completed before the challenge. If things have become more positive for you, that's awesome! Why do you think this is? Is it because your life has changed an awful lot in the last ten days? It might have budged a little, but it's likely more to with your perspective and resilience. In other words, it's probably about how well you mentally digest what's going on around you.

If your ratings haven't shifted at all, or maybe even gone in the wrong direction (the horror!), think about why that might be. Have you approached the challenge from a mindset of thinking you're not good enough to change? Are you stuck in a cycle that needs a professional therapist's outside view? If you think you might need mental health therapy but are a bit hesitant, think of it as just like rehab exercises after knee surgery. You have to go and see the specialist regularly to make sure the exercises are working.

If you did the challenge half-arsed and didn't complete your daily non-negotiables, I beg you, please do them and restart the challenge. If you think they seem like airy nonsense, have a look at some of the science (listed in the references) about why they can help you. If you don't fancy doing them even after I've literally begged you to, go ahead and do the challenges again if you want to, but know that you're not getting the most out of them.

Don't beat yourself up if you slip back into old habits or feel like you forget what you learned through this exercise. Just pick up the book and remind yourself, or have a flick through the notes you've made yourself as part of the daily non-negotiables and daily challenges. Life isn't about being perfect, or being happy all the time. Happiness is about resilience, and rising to challenges with the sense that you can overcome what gets thrown at you...or that you can at least catch it before it hits you in the face.

CHALLENGE SUMMARY

If you've read the book in its entirety (of course) and just need a quick reference point for doing the daily challenges, you're welcome:

Preparation: Rate your life. Get hold of a notebook to start writing in.

Daily non-negotiables: Diarise the time to every day write down three gratitudes, three ways you've ever made someone's life better (positive impacts), and do ten minutes of mindfulness OR 20 mins exercise.

Day 1: Compliments - give a sincere, genuine, well thought-out compliment to at least one person, but preferably three different people.

Day 2: Connect with someone important - call a friend or family member, arrange to see them or arrange a video call with them. Or start a community project, volunteer to hang out (in person or online) with an elderly person who needs the company even more than you do.

Day 3: Make your world a better place. Contribute time, money or goods to an organisation that you believe in.

Day 4: Sustainability breeds contentment – engage in behaviours that lessen or negate your impact on the planet.

Day 5: Meaningful work – two to three actions from a long list of options that bring purpose to your day job.

Day 6: Use your sadness to your advantage - acknowledge, label and reframe a negative thought process.

Day 7: Hobbies – take an interest in something new.

Day 8: Exercise! 20 minutes extra is all it takes.

Day 9: Use your gratitudes – read them, share them, enjoy them. Praise yourself for your positive impacts and appreciate what you've achieved in your life so far.

Day 10: Plan your routine from now on, and whether to repeat the whole challenge over again. Repeat 2 of the daily challenges to finish off with a bang. Repeat your ratings and reflect on what happened over the course of the last 10 days. Have a look at your goals and see if you're on your way towards them.

Don't forget to congratulate yourself on the effort you've put in, not necessarily the short term outcome, like a true realistic optimist. You don't need to have done everything perfectly to have still made a good effort, and to have begun the process of updating your mindset. Enjoy that process, and remember that the only person who can control your happiness, is the one reading this book.

REFERENCES

(In   order   of   appearance)

Goyal, M et al (2013) Meditation programs for psychological stress and well-being: a systematic review and meta-analysis. JAMA Intern Med. 2014 Mar;174(3):357-68.   doi: 10.1001/jamainternmed.2013.13018.

Toepfer, S.M., Cichy, K. & Peters, P. (2012) Letters of Gratitude: Further Evidence for Author Benefits. J Happiness   Stud   13:   187–201 https://doi.org/10.1007/s10902-011-9257-7

Day   1:

Sugawara SK et al (2012) Social Rewards Enhance Offline Improvements in Motor Skill. PLoS ONE 7(11): e48174. https://doi.org/10.1371/journal.pone.0048174

Izuma, K et al (2008) Processing of Social and Monetary Rewards in the Human Striatum J Neuron 58(2):284-294 https://doi.org/10.1016/j.neuron.2008.03.020 Bedosky, R et al (2018) The Psychology of Giving and Receiving Compliments J Happiness Studies, 7(3), 361-375

Achor, S (2016) The Benefits of Peer-to-Peer Praise at Work   Harvard   Business   Review http://www.shawnachor.com/harvard-business-review-the-benefits-of-peer-to-peer-praise-at-work/

Day   2:

Waldinger RJ, Schulz MS. What's love got to do with it? Social functioning, perceived health, and daily happiness in married octogenarians. Psychol Aging. 2010;25(2):422–431.   doi:10.1037/a0019087

Sandstrom GM, Dunn EW.(2014) Social Interactions and Well-Being: The Surprising Power of Weak Ties. Pers Soc Psychol   Bull.   40(7):910–922. doi:10.1177/0146167214529799

Day   3:

Larson, R. (1989). Is Feeling "in Control" Related to Happiness in Daily Life? Psychological Reports, 64(3), 775–784.

The Life You Can Save - www.thelifeyoucansave.org Change Path - www.changepath.com Myer, D.G. The Secrets of Happiness Psychology Today. 1992. (https://www.psychologytoday.com/articles/200910/the-secrets-happiness)

Whillans AV, Dunn EW, Smeets P, Bekkers R, Norton MI. Buying time promotes happiness. Proc Natl Acad Sci U S A. 2017;114(32):8523–8527. doi:10.1073/pnas.1706541114

Dunn, E et al (2008) Spending Money on Others Promotes Happiness Science 319(5870): 1687-1688

Matz SC, Gladstone JJ, Stillwell D. Money Buys Happiness When Spending Fits Our Personality. Psychol Sci. 2016;27(5):715–725.

Day 4:

Kasser, T (2005) Are Psychological and Ecological Wellbeing Compatible? The Role of Values, Mindfulness and Lifestyle. Social Indicators Research 74:349-368

Coral-Verdugo, V et al (2011) Happiness as Correlate of Sustainable Behavior: A Study of Pro-Ecological, Frugal, Equitable and Altruistic Actions That Promote Subjective Wellbeing. Res in Human Ecology 18(2):95-104

Landes, X et al (2015) Sustainable Happiness: Why Waste Prevention May Lead to an Increase in Quality of Life. The Happiness Research Institute Report.

Day 5:

Ferguson, D (2015) The World's Happiest Jobs for The Guardian Newspaper https://www.theguardian.com/money/2015/apr/07/going-to-work-with-a-smile-on-your-face Krog Norgoord G et al (2016) The Job Satisfaction Index. The Happiness Research Institute and Krifa

Day 6:

Erskine JA, Georgiou GJ (2010) Effects of thought

suppression on eating behaviour in restrained and non-restrained eaters. Appetite. 54(3):499–503. doi:10.1016/j.appet.2010.02.001

Bryant RA, Wyzenbeek M, Weinstein J. Dream rebound of suppressed emotional thoughts: the influence of cognitive load. Conscious Cogn. 2011;20(3):515–522. doi:10.1016/j.concog.2010.11.004

Garland E.L., Roberts-Lewis, A (2013) Differential roles of thought suppression and dispositional mindfulness in posttraumatic stress symptoms and craving. Addictive Behaviours 38:1555–1562

Kroner-Borowick, T et al (2013) The effects of suppressing intrusive thoughts on dream content, dream distress and psychological parameters. J Sleep Res. 22:600–604

Adler JM, Hershfield HE. Mixed emotional experience is associated with and precedes improvements in psychological well-being. PLoS One. 2012;7(4):e35633. doi:10.1371/journal.pone.0035633

Day 7: Walikzeck, TM et al (2005) The Influence of Gardening Activities on Consumer Perceptions of Life Satisfaction. Hort Science 40 (5) 1360-1365

Brooks L, Ta KN, Townsend AF, Backman CL. (2019) "I just love it": Avid knitters describe health and well-being through occupation. Can J Occup Ther. 86(2):114–124. doi:10.1177/0008417419831401

Beiser M, Feldman JJ, Egelhoff CJ. Assets and affects. A study of positive mental health. Arch Gen Psychiatry. 1972;27(4):545–549. doi:10.1001/archpsyc.1972.01750280103017

Lu L, Argyle M. Leisure satisfaction and happiness as a function of leisure activity. Gaoxiong Yi Xue Ke Xue Za Zhi. 1994;10(2):89–96.

Day 8: Loprinzi, PD, Cardinal, BJ (2011) Association between objectively-measured physical activity and sleep, NHANES 2005–2006. J Mental Health and Physical Activity 4(2)65-69

Burton, J.P., Hoobler, J.M. & Scheuer, M.L. (2012) Supervisor Workplace Stress and Abusive Supervision: The Buffering Effect of Exercise. J Bus Psychol 27: 271–279. https://doi.org/10.1007/s10869-011-9255-0

Pasco JA, Jacka FN, Williams LJ, Brennan SL, Leslie E, Berk M. (2011) Don't worry, be active: positive affect and habitual physical activity. Aust N Z J Psychiatry 45(12):1047–1052.

Coulson, JC et al (2008) Exercising at work and self-reported work performance in International Journal of Workplace Health Management 1(3):176-197

Hackney AC, Lane AR, Register-Mihalik J, O'leary CB (2017) Endurance Exercise Training and Male Sexual Libido. Med Sci Sports Exerc. 49(7):1383–1388.

Weggemans RM, Backx FJG, Borghouts L, et al. (2018) The 2017 Dutch Physical Activity Guidelines. Int J Behav Nutr Phys Act.15(1):58. Published 2018 Jun 25. Day 9:

Hernandez R, Kershaw KN, Siddique J, et al. (2015) Optimism and Cardiovascular Health: Multi-Ethnic Study of Atherosclerosis (MESA). Health Behav Policy Rev. 2015;2(1):62–73. doi:10.14485/HBPR.2.1.6

Kim ES, Hagan KA, Grodstein F, DeMeo DL, De Vivo I, Kubzansky LD. (2017) Optimism and Cause-Specific Mortality: A Prospective Cohort Study. Am J Epidemiol.185(1):21–29. doi:10.1093/aje/kww182

Jefferson A, Bortolotti L, Kuzmanovic B. (2017) What is unrealistic optimism?. Conscious Cogn. 50:3–11. doi:10.1016/j.concog.2016.10.005 Chou, S (2013) Realistic optimism presentation to American Psychological Association, Honolulu Aug 2013.

Wimberly SR, Carver CS, Antoni MH. Effects of optimism, interpersonal relationships, and distress on psychosexual well-being among women with early stage breast cancer. Psychol Health. 2008;23(1):57–72. doi:10.1080/14768320701204211

De Neve JE, Oswald AJ. Estimating the influence of life

satisfaction and positive affect on later income using sibling fixed effects. Proc Natl Acad Sci U S A. 2012;109(49):19953–19958. doi:10.1073/pnas.1211437109

Stavrova O, Ehlebracht D. Cynical beliefs about human nature and income: Longitudinal and cross-cultural analyses. J Pers Soc Psychol. 2016;110(1):116–132. doi:10.1037/pspp0000050

Stavrova O. Having a Happy Spouse Is Associated With Lowered Risk of Mortality. Psychol Sci. 2019;30(5):798–803.   doi:10.1177/0956797619835147

ABOUT THE AUTHOR

Anna Brown is a self-confessed science nerd, with an interest in all things happiness. As a health professional in the 21st century, it's come to her attention that a person's health is not about just one particular approach, but is determined by their entire daily life and experience of the world. Watching current events unfold, Anna believes that now, more than ever, we need to build a resilient, optimistic, healthy society.

www.ingramcontent.com/pod-product-compliance
Lightning Source LLC
Chambersburg PA
CBHW060720030426
42337CB00017B/2935